PROTEIN -

A Secret to

Losing Weight?

Why (and How) Protein Helps You Drop Those Pounds

RON KNESS

Contents

Disclaimer

This publication is for informational purposes only and is not intended as medical advice. Medical advice should always be obtained from a qualified medical professional for any health conditions or symptoms associated with them.

Every possible effort has been made in preparing and researching this material. We make no warranties with respect to the accuracy, applicability of its contents or any omissions.

See your healthcare professional before starting any diet, health or exercise program!

Introduction

Protein, carbohydrates and fats are essential to your existence. Those are the 3 macronutrients found in your food that the body requires in large amounts, and must continually be replaced. If you don't get sufficient quantities of those nutrients in the foods you eat, a host of medical problems and health issues will develop. And while a lot has been written about carbohydrates and fats, in regard to losing weight, very little is written on how protein can help you drop those pounds too.

As a structural component of tissue which makes up your muscles, hair, skin, enzymes and antibodies, protein is required by every cell in the human body. It helps your body grow and repair cells, and is absolutely essential for cellular activity. Periods of intense growth, such as infancy, childhood and pregnancy, require more protein than usual, and if you are injured, recovering from surgery or stay active, you also need more protein than you normally would.

Did you know your body can actually make protein?

While there are hundreds of microscopic compounds called amino acids in nature, your body only benefits from 22 of them. Of those 22, humans can't produce 9 of those essential acids. They must be obtained by eating food.

So, just eat a lot of protein and you will stay healthy, right? The answer to that question is yes... and no. Your body can only absorb and use a specific amount of protein at any given time.

Just like all of the compounds in the food you eat and the beverages you drink, if you take in too much, the excess gets passed out as waste.

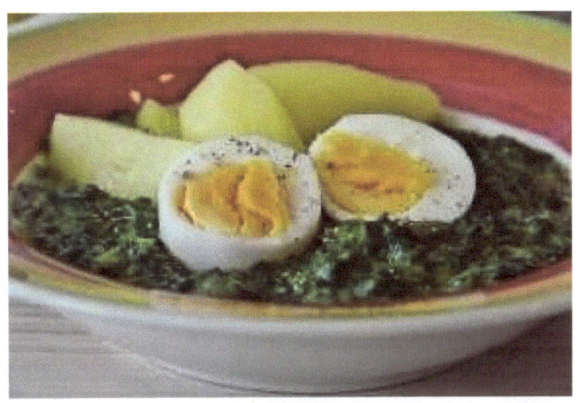

This is why it is better for your health to consume your daily protein requirement spread out over 3 or 4 meals, rather than trying to get it all at once. As it turns out, getting several daily doses of protein is an eating behavior that can help you lose weight if you are overweight, and it also helps you stay at your target weight once you get there.

In this book, we will take an in-depth look at the weight loss/protein relationship. You will discover just how much protein health authorities say you should be getting every day, and what happens when you eat too much.

You will find out which healthy foods are protein-rich, and you may just be surprised at some of the foods on this list. You'll get the lowdown on protein bars, powders and shakes, why the "when" of eating protein is so important, and how you should time your protein consumption to get the most out of your workout.

Let's get started by taking a look at how your body processes protein, and how this can result in weight loss.

How Does Protein Help You Lose Weight?

Once, a very long time ago, you did not know how to ride a bike. You saw other kids riding their bikes, and you longed to join them in their experience of freedom and independence. You started out with training wheels, and slowly taught your body how to move, the exact process of coordination needed for you to stay on your bike.

You eventually took off the training wheels, learned to ride on just two wheels, and now you don't have to give a second thought to riding a bicycle. It has become second nature. Just as riding a bicycle is a specific process, the way your body removes protein from food and uses it to keep you strong and healthy is a process as well.

When you eat food, it works its way through your digestive tract. It goes into your mouth, travels down your throat and esophagus and into your stomach. Once there, powerful stomach acids and enzymes begin to break down your food. One of those enzymes is pepsin, and pepsin's favorite "food" is protein. Pepsin breaks down the peptide bonds which hold protein molecules together.

Once this happens, protein moves into your small intestine, where it is further digested by pancreatic enzymes such as chymotrypsin, trypsin and carboxypeptidase. Then protein is broken down into amino acids, the building blocks of the human body. Once protein is chiseled down to amino acids, they are transported into your bloodstream, and then delivered to every part of your body.

This process takes a while.

It can take as many as 1.5 hours for your body to process a protein shake so that amino acids can be absorbed into your bloodstream. Solid food sources of protein can take even longer to process. This is because the 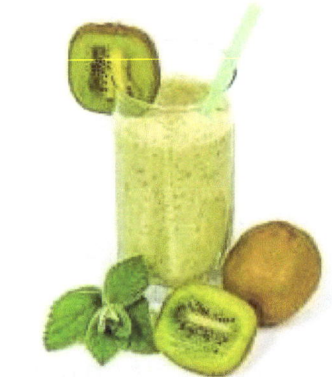 presence of protein in your digestive system triggers the release of a hormone that slows down how fast your stomach empties its contents.

The longer it takes to process a particular food in your body means the longer you can keep hunger at bay.

In weightlifting, bodybuilding, fitness and medical communities, there is a constant debate as to the exact rate of speed your body breaks down and absorbs protein. What is not debated is that there is a substantial time requirement. This process also slows down the contractions of your intestines that help digest your food, which is why you feel full longer after eating protein-rich foods than you do carbohydrates and fats.

This helps reduce your appetite. Eat protein at every meal, and you will consume fewer calories overall, since your body will be spending much of the day processing protein and keeping you feeling full.

This is great news. It means that the act of digesting protein speeds up your metabolic process. The energy for breaking protein down into amino acids, called thermogenics, requires a lot of fuel. That fuel comes from calories, fats and carbohydrates. Protein is also excellent for building muscle. The more muscle you have, the more fat you burn, because muscles require a lot of fuel to maintain and repair themselves, and that fuel is the same fats, calories and carbohydrates which the protein-digesting formula requires.

Now you know exactly why a protein-rich diet is recommended by so many health and wellness professionals for healthy weight loss, and weight regulation.

Is There Such a Thing as Too Much Protein?

Your body is made up predominantly of water. Water is essential to human existence. If you went without getting any water into your body, you would not live more than just about 3 days. While this is obviously a very important human need, if you ingest too much water too quickly, you can drown. As far as protein is concerned, getting too much can have a negative effect as well.

Excessive protein on a regular basis has been linked to health problems as insignificant as nausea and diarrhea, and even life-threatening conditions caused by excess amino acids, insulin and ammonia. So it is wise to know exactly how much protein you should be consuming every day. Here are a few recommendations from some respected health authorities.

The Mayo Clinic suggests "5 to 6 ounces of protein-rich food each day". This could deliver anywhere from 50 to 70 grams (g) of protein, and is only meant as a suggestion for someone who is normally active, with a healthy body weight.

The Institute of Medicine in the United States publishes what they call the Dietary Reference Intake, or DRI. In it they suggest eating "0.8 grams of protein per kilogram of body weight, or 0.36 g per pound" every day.

The Reference Nutrient Intake (RNI) of the UK's National Health Service suggests 0.75 g for each kilogram of body weight, or 0.34 g per pound.

Since eating too much protein or not enough can cause health problems, a "Protein Summit" was convened in Washington, DC in 2015. More than 40 nutrition scientists focused on how protein affects human health.

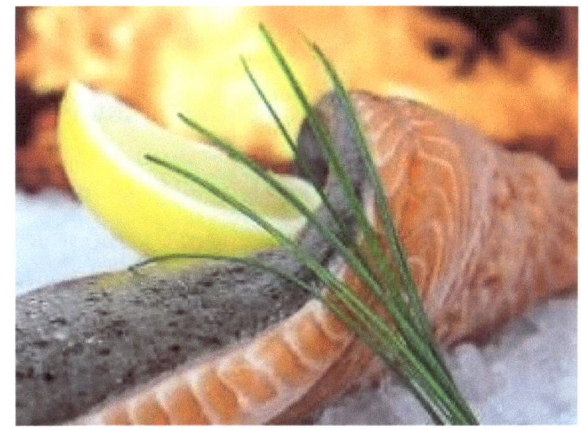

Their findings were reported in a supplemental issue of the **American Journal of Clinical Nutrition** (AJCN). What those nutrition experts found is that most Americans are not eating anywhere near enough protein.

For slowing down the aging process, losing weight, building muscle and supporting cardiovascular health, they recommend eating protein as a source of 15% to 25% of your daily calories. They went on to say that if you got as much as 35% of your daily calories from protein, you would probably not suffer any ill effects.

All of the above recommendations are for someone who is mildly active. If you follow a healthy exercise regimen regularly, you want to up your protein intake. As mentioned earlier, the same is true if you are pregnant or recovering from an illness or surgery.

Can Protein Make You Fat?

Okay, so you know how much protein you should be getting into your body every day. You also know that spreading your protein intake out over the course of the day is easier on your digestive system, and can boost your weight loss efforts. Since protein is required by every cell in your body, getting plenty of this nutrient can lead to multiple health benefits. However, too much of a good thing can often become a bad thing.

That's the case with protein, which your body sometimes turns into fat.

Just like the fat and carbohydrates we discussed earlier, protein provides calories. When you get an excess amount of protein in your body, it is converted into glycogen and then glucose, providing a caloric source of energy. When your body has more energy than it needs, it is converted into body fat.

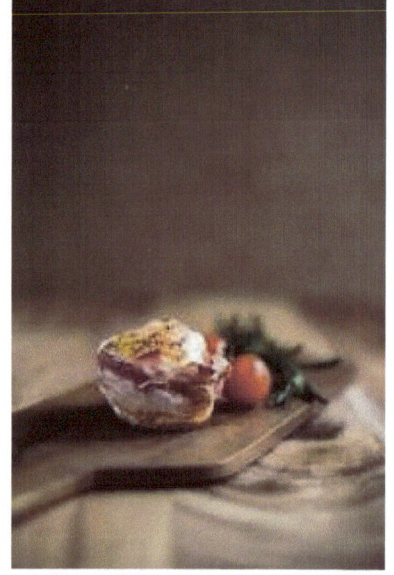

As you probably know, when you are heavier than your ideal weight, you put stress and strain on your joints, your heart, your kidneys and other body parts. You raise your risk of diabetes and cancer dramatically when you become overweight or obese.

What can you do to ensure you are not endangering yourself by eating too much protein? Keep a food journal. Chronicle every piece of food that goes into your body, along with your physical characteristics and experiences.

Figure out your daily calorie intake, and what percent of that is protein. Monitor the results, and make changes accordingly. If you stay within the 10% to 25% range of daily calories from protein, studies show that is a healthy place to be.

Making the Most of Your Workouts with Protein

You will often hear bodybuilders talk about eating protein before and after a workout. Other athletes do the same. Health and fitness experts will tell you the human body burns calories and fat, and repairs muscle, for up to 48 hours after you exercise. Since protein speeds up your metabolism and builds muscle so well, you need to structure your workouts to include some type of protein source.

Bear in mind that everyone is different. Your body is unique in so many ways. Your metabolism will work slower or faster than others, and the way your system processes protein may be quicker or slower than the norm. In general terms, however, the following tips on when to add protein to your exercise will probably lead to the best results.

Science shows that food sources of protein are harder to break down than liquids. This means you should allow 1 or 2 hours before your workout plans to consume solid sources of protein. A protein shake or drink is absorbed quickly, so you could opt for drinking one 30 minutes before you exercise.

Immediately following a workout or exercise program, or if you just burned up the dance floor, you should get protein into your body. This is the time-frame when your system utilizes protein at its very best. Eating 10 to 20 g of protein within 15 to 30 minutes after you are physically active is recommended by many health and fitness experts.

Don't forget to stay hydrated before, during and after any type of physical activity. Drink 16 ounces of water within 2 hours of exercising, and hydrate afterwards as well. A hydrated body is necessary to effectively break down and absorb protein.

Be Careful About Which Protein You Choose Post Workout

When you want to lose weight and build muscle mass, you not only improve your health, but you improve your posture, the way that your body can move, your stamina and you even gain more energy.

After working out, there's a lot of advice that will tell you that

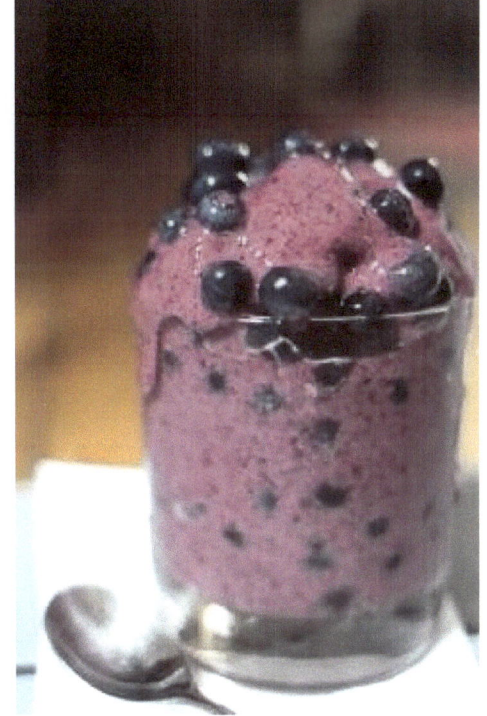

it's best for you to get some protein in your system. Since no one wants to down a full meal (including protein) right after finishing up a workout, what most people do is reach for something quick and convenient that's loaded with protein.

For some people that's a protein bar. For others, that's a protein shake. After all, if it's loaded with protein, it has to be good for you, right?

Maybe. But then again, maybe not.

The foods that you choose after your workout might not be the best ones for you. In fact, they might actually be working to hinder your weight loss efforts. Many of the protein foods or drinks that you can get for use after a workout concentrate on building muscle rather than weight loss.

This means that you have to pay attention to the label. Some of them are going to have more than twice the amount of calories and protein level that you really need.

Stick to the protein that's best for your weight loss if that's your goal. However, if you want to build muscle mass while losing weight, then you're going to want to choose the protein product that helps you with that goal.

The protein food for after your workout should also be in line with the amount of exercise you're performing during it. The harder you work out, the more protein that you need.

One of the ways that your protein choice might not be so good for you is found in the type of sweetener the product contains. You can find some with real sugar and some with artificial sweeteners.

While the artificial ones are often sweeter than sugar and don't give you the same high calorie content, artificial sweeteners aren't right for everyone. When selecting a protein food for after your workout, look for those that are high in taste quality but lower in sugar.

Pay attention to ingredient lists that have a lot of milk content or nut butters because these can pile on the sugar. Make sure that if you use protein powder that it has quality ingredients and isn't heavier on the carbs than it is the protein.

Watch out for powders that have a lot of unnecessary ingredients. If you do choose protein powder, it should have at least 20 grams of protein per serving. To get the most from your protein choice, make sure you consume it within 60 minutes of your workout so that your muscles get the most benefit.

The Best Sources of Healthy Protein for Weight Loss

Excessive amounts of protein can aggravate liver or kidney conditions. If you plan on significantly upping the amount of protein in your diet, speak to your physician first. Once you and your health team decide how much protein will give you the best weight loss benefits, focus on getting more of your protein from the following sources:

- Seafood, wild-caught instead of farm-raised

- Beans

- Lean meats, grass-fed instead of grain-fed

- Low-fat dairy and eggs, pasture-raised and organic if possible

- Nuts and seeds

These protein-filled foods are full of nutrients and vitamins, and lower in saturated fat than some other foods. You can also benefit in your weight loss and health improvement efforts by constantly eating different types of food that contain protein. For instance, beans are full of healthy dietary fiber and salmon is an excellent source of the omega-3 essential fatty acids your body craves.

Different protein sources promote different health characteristics. Eat several of the foods just mentioned throughout the day to give your body the best chance at benefiting from protein.

It should be noted that you cannot process more than about 20 g of protein at a time. Remember this when planning your meals, as eating more protein than that at a single time creates unnecessary waste, and doesn't help your pocketbook either.

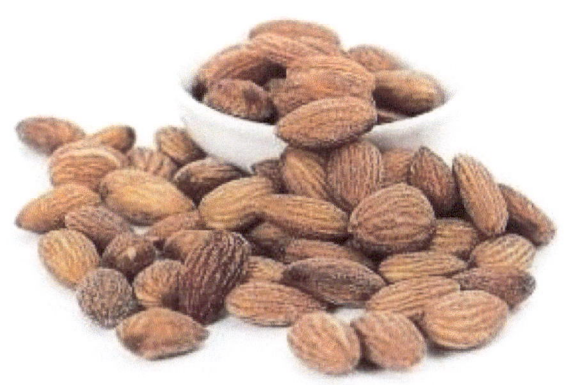

Do Veggies and Fruit Have Any Protein?

Vegetarians and meat eaters don't agree on much where diet is concerned. One thing they definitely do agree on is the importance of protein for a healthy body. However, meat eaters will say that you simply can't get enough protein into your body on a regular basis from vegetables, fruits, nuts, beans and a predominantly plant-based diet.

Vegetarians will tell you differently.

So many vegetarians and vegans live to a rather ripe old age eating nothing but plants. This is because significant protein is found in many foods.

The following list tells you how much of certain plant-based foods you need to eat to get a specific amount of protein into your body.

- Sprouted beans, peas and lentils – 8 to 10 g of protein per cup

- Cooked lima beans – 11 to 12 g of protein per cup

- Green peas – 7 to 8 g of protein per cup

- Cooked succotash, a mixture of lima beans and corn – 9 and 10 g of protein per cup

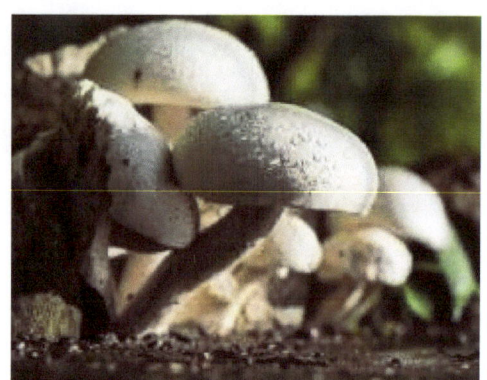

- White mushrooms, cooked – 4 g of protein per cup, sliced

- Yellow sweet corn – 4 to 5 g of protein per cup

- Globe artichokes – 4 grams of protein per artichoke

- Cooked spinach – 5 g of protein per cup

- Cooked collard greens – 1 g of protein per cup

- Cooked mustard greens – 1.5 grams of protein per cup

- Broccoli – 2.5 to 3 grams of protein per cup chopped

- Brussels sprouts cooked – 4 g of protein per cup

- Cooked asparagus – 4 to 4.5 grams of protein per cup

- Kale - 1 gram of protein per cup

- Nuts – 6 g per 2-ounce serving

There are significantly higher levels of protein in meat and other animal-based foods than there usually is in fruits and vegetables. Eating even small amounts of the following foods can deliver large amounts of protein.

- Steak, bottom or top round – 23 g of protein per 3 ounces

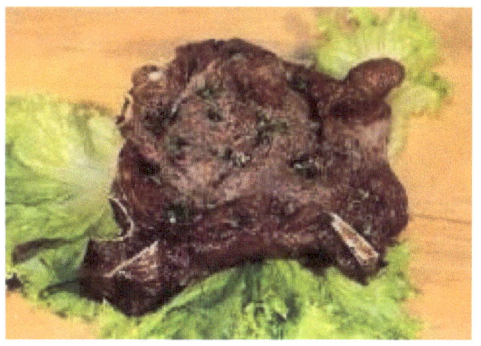

- Ribeye steak – 14 g of protein per 3 ounces

- 95% lean ground beef – 18 g protein per 3-ounce serving

- Boneless pork chops – 26 g per 3 ounces

- Boneless, skinless chicken breast – 24 g per 3 ounces

- Turkey breast – 24 g per 3 ounces

- Sockeye salmon – 23 g per 3 ounces

- Sardines – 21 g per 3 ounces

- Light tuna – 22 g per 3 ounces

- Canned chicken – 21 g per 3 ounces

- Navy beans – 20 g per 1 cup serving

- Greek yogurt – 23 g of protein per 8-ounce serving

- Swiss cheese – 8 g per 1-ounce slice or serving

- Cottage cheese – 14 g per 1/2 cup serving

- Eggs – 6 g per large egg

Final Thoughts

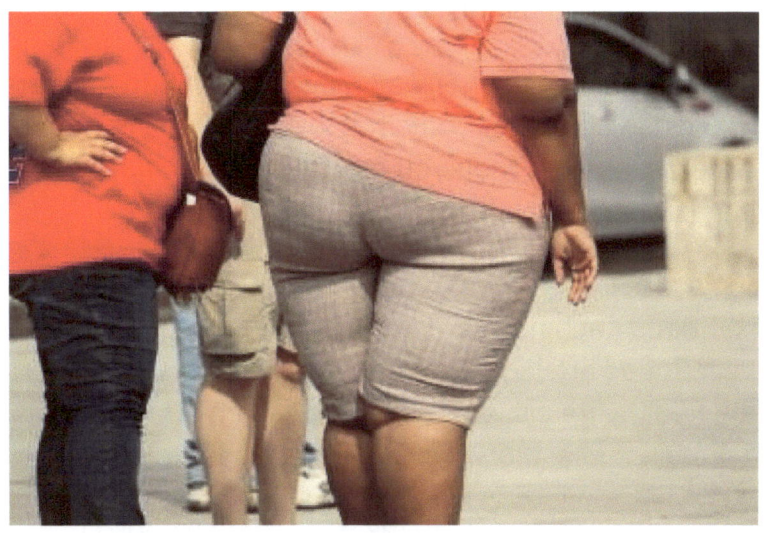

Obesity in America has risen to levels that are at an all-time high. Not only has this weight epidemic struck adults, but children as well. This health condition makes everyone a target for developing diseases like diabetes, coronary disease, and even certain cancers.

But your diet can change all of that - especially if it's one that's filled with protein. There are many diets on the market that promote eating a lot of protein. As it turns out, those diets were definitely on the right track.

When you consume a diet that's rich in protein it actually does help you lose weight. There's a scientific reason why your body likes you eating protein and responds with weight loss.

When you eat a diet that's high in protein, it helps your appetite slow down. You get a natural appetite suppressor by eating protein. Eating protein causes your body to create an amino acid that makes you lose weight.

This acid is known as phenylalanine. This, in turn, triggers the response from your body that tells you that your appetite has been satiated. When you feel full, you don't end up eating as much.

Eating a diet that's high in protein is a lot easier than you think. Foods each have a different amount of protein. Some of these foods are higher in protein than others, but if you create healthy meals where the focus is on filling your plate with protein items, then you're going to lose weight.

You can snack on protein items, too - such as boiled eggs, which are high in protein - or have some cubed chicken breast, which also has a lot of protein. Each time you eat foods that contain protein, your body produces the phenylalanine.

In studies conducted on how this affects weight loss efforts, it was shown that subjects given phenylalanine had higher levels of GLP-1. This is a natural way of controlling your appetite as well as lowering the amount of hormones that make you feel hungry.

Not only did the phenylalanine in the test subjects help them lose weight, but it also helped them be more physically active. Even better news is that when studies were done on test subjects that were obese, the ones given phenylalanine also lost weight.

It worked by specifically directing its focus on the CaSR, which is a receptor in the body that's used to lower your appetite. The results of these new studies can be used to help stop the rising tide of obesity and help those currently dealing with the issue to successfully lose weight.

Protein for Weight Loss Checklist

Protein is essential, no matter what your fitness goals are. For weight loss, just staying in shape or to build massive amounts of muscle and 6-pack abs, protein is an absolute necessity. Here are some protein tips to keep in mind for weight loss, and they also support overall health and well-being.

☐ Your body can only process a small amount of protein at a time, roughly 20 grams (g). This means you should spread protein out across all your meals, rather than eating one large amount of protein at any single meal.

☐ There are significantly higher levels of protein in animal-based foods than plant-based foods. A 3-ounce serving of steak delivers anywhere from 14 to 23 g of protein.

☐ It is possible to get all of your protein requirements fulfilled by eating plants only. Lima beans offer 11 to 12 g of protein per cup, and just 2 ounces of nuts get 6 g of protein into your body.

☐ Whey protein powder delivers what is called a "complete protein". This is because it contains all 9 of the amino acids the human body requires, but cannot produce itself.

☐ Eat protein for breakfast and you may eat fewer calories throughout the day. That fact is supported by a study which showed that consuming 20 g of protein at breakfast led to a drop in how many calories were eaten the rest of the day.

☐ If you eat too much protein, it can be stored as fat.

☐ The Mayo Clinic suggests eating 5 to 6 ounces of protein-rich food each day.

☐ US and UK health officials recommend eating around 0.80 g of protein per kilogram of body weight daily, or roughly 0.35 grams per pound.

☐ Many global health organizations agree that eating protein that equals 15% to 25% of your daily calories is a healthy move.

☐ Eat solid protein food sources 1 to 2 hours before you work out. If you choose a protein shake or powder instead, 30 minutes before you exercise is best.

☐ Estimates vary, but it is generally agreed that eating 10 to 20 g of protein 15 to 30 minutes after you exercise offers the most benefits.

☐ Some healthy sources of protein include fish and seafood (caught in the wild, not farm-raised), nuts and seeds, beans and lean meats, and low-fat dairy and eggs.

☐ A large egg has about 6 g of protein. This is considered by health experts to be a "perfect protein", and is one reason why eggs are considered superfoods.

Plant-Based vs. Animal Based Protein Checklist

Protein is required by every cell in your body. It helps your muscles repair and heal so they grow strong and healthy, it influences how every one of your physiological processes works, and can help you reach any number of fitness goals. That is why it is so important to get the recommended 0.80 grams of protein per kilogram of body weight (0.36 g per pound) into your body every day.

Protein is found in a diverse variety of foods. There is protein in eggs, nuts, kale, steak, chicken and seafood. Whether you decide to eat plant or animal-based foods to get your protein is up to you. The following two lists can help you choose.

No matter what type protein-rich food you enjoy, opt for organic, pastured-raised, grass-fed and wild-caught as opposed to processed whenever you can.

Plant-Based Protein

- Sprouted beans, peas and lentils – 8 to 10 g of protein per cup

- Cooked lima beans – 11 to 12 g of protein per cup

- Green peas – 7 to 8 g of protein per cup

- Cooked succotash, a mixture of lima beans and corn

– 9 and 10 g of protein per cup

- White mushrooms, cooked – 4 g of protein per cup, sliced

- Yellow sweet corn – 4 to 5 g of protein per cup

- Globe artichokes – 4 grams of protein per artichoke

- Cooked spinach – 5 g of protein per cup

- Cooked collard greens – 1 g of protein per cup

- Cooked mustard greens – 1.5 grams of protein per cup

- Broccoli – 2.5 to 3 grams of protein per cup chopped

- Brussels sprouts cooked – 4 g of protein per cup

- Cooked asparagus – 4 to 4.5 grams of protein per cup

- Kale - 1 gram of protein per cup

- Nuts – 6 g per 2-ounce serving

Animal-Based Protein

- Steak, bottom or top round – 23 g of protein per 3 ounces

- Ribeye steak – 14 g of protein per 3 ounces

- 95% lean ground beef – 18 g protein per 3-ounce serving

- Boneless pork chops – 26 g per 3 ounces

- Boneless, skinless chicken breast – 24 g per 3 ounces

- Turkey breast – 24 g per 3 ounces

- Sockeye salmon – 23 g per 3 ounces

- Sardines – 21 g per 3 ounces

- Light tuna – 22 g per 3 ounces

- Canned chicken – 21 g per 3 ounces

- Navy beans – 20 g per 1 cup serving

- Greek yogurt – 23 g of protein per 8-ounce serving

- Swiss cheese – 8 g per 1-ounce slice or serving

- Cottage cheese – 14 g per 1/2 cup serving

Other Relevant Books by This Author

If you would like to read more relevant books about this topic, here is a list of the CreateSpace links, titles and descriptions from this author:

https://www.createspace.com/6758654

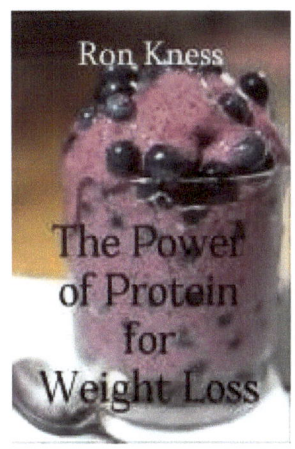

The Power of Protein for Weight Loss: Accelerate Weight Loss With Protein

Anyone who has ever tried to lose weight knows that there are ups and downs, ebbs and flows.

Some people get frustrated and stop trying to lose weight because they go on these complicated diets that either introduce foods that are as appetizing as cardboard or they strictly limit foods they love.

Not only is that not appealing and not healthy for the body, but it doesn't lead to long term, successful weight loss. One of the simplest ways to lose weight is to make sure you're getting the protein that your body needs.

If you're eliminating or severely limiting protein, or simply not paying attention to the fact that you're loading up on carbs and ignoring the protein aspect, then it could be one of the reasons why your weight loss journey has been a struggle.

Your body was made to need protein. You need it from head to toe. The cells throughout your body have to have it. Without enough protein, you'll end up with thinning hair and weak nails.

Your body will struggle to stay healthy - to keep your muscles and tissues in good working order. You'll suffer from a lack of certain hormones and you can damage your bones without having enough protein in your diet.

But a huge reason that you need to eat protein might surprise you. You need protein because it gives you energy. And energy is what enables you to be able to do whatever it is that you need to do throughout the day.

Lack of protein is a big reason why so many diets people have tried, fail. Who cares what foods you eat when you're so tired and so drained that all you want to do is collapse on the sofa and not move?

Diets that don't include a focus on protein will eventually wear you out and you won't want to stick to them. And you shouldn't. You need protein to give you the right amount of energy that will sustain you all the way through your journey to weight loss success.

Let me show you how to get enough protein in your diet and how protein helps you with your weight loss efforts.

https://www.createspace.com/4963196

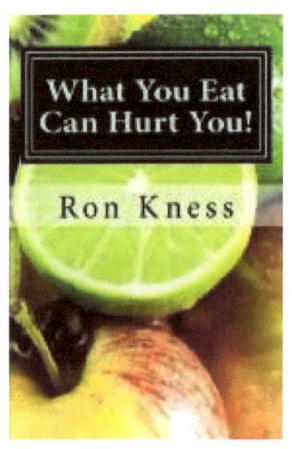

What You Eat Can Hurt You!: Learn Which Foods to Avoid and Which Ones to Eat to Stamp Out Inflammation, Illness and Disease, and to Stay Healthy!

Do you know that certain foods increase your risk for inflammation, disease and illness? It's true! And certain foods can help cure and heal you if you do get sick. Knowing which foods to eat and which ones to avoid empowers you to manage your own health.

After all, you have to look out for yourself.

Other topics discussed in this book are:
==> Health Mismanagement in Today's Society
==> Boost Your Health the Natural Way
==> Fight Disease with Proper Nutrition
==> Diabetic Nutritional Management
==> Prevent and Reverse Heart Disease the Natural Way
==> Take a Bite Out of Inflammation With Food
==> Remember, Nutrition Boosts Your Memory
==> News Flash - Control and Cure Cancer Through Nutrition
==> How to Cook Healthy

Take charge of your health today and learn which foods will keep you healthy and heal you, and which ones can make you sick or slow your healing. Click on the Buy Now with One Click button now and start reading in minutes how to maintain your health or get well.

https://www.createspace.com/6345319

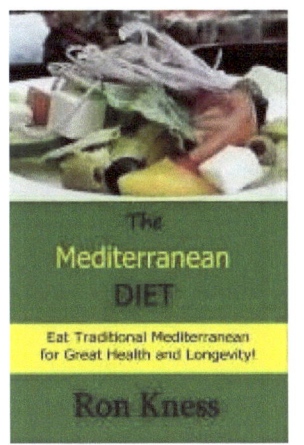

The Mediterranean Diet: Eat Traditional Mediterranean for Great Health and Longevity!

The Mediterranean Diet is one of the very best diets there is for anyone who wants to lose weight in a way that's healthy, fun and sustainable. This is a diet that's all about treating food with respect and all about getting natural ingredients in a way that you can actually enjoy.

And the benefits of that are incredible. The numbers speak for themselves but it goes beyond just lifespan and heart health. This is a diet that can make you feel the best you've felt in years.

Somewhere along the way, our approach to diet here in the US has become twisted. I'm talking about our general diet sure but I'm also talking about our attempts to eat healthily and lose weight! And in many ways, our diet is a reflection of our lifestyle: everything is fast, convenient and consumable. At the same time though, it lacks substance and it lacks passion.

We have lost respect for our diet and we've stopped seeing food as something to be enjoyed. Instead, we see it as an inconvenience. We're too busy to eat – and so we grab the quickest thing to eat from the cupboard or the fridge. Normally that means eating ready-made meals that are full of sugar and processed meats, or it means eating Mars Bars that literally offer us zero nutrition.
Unsurprisingly, this leads to many of us gaining a lot of weight as all we're eating is sugar and in high quantities.

At the same time, our skin, hair and nails look damaged because we aren't getting the bioavailable amino acids or the vitamins and minerals that we need. All that sugar has led to an epidemic of diabetes and many other preventable diseases are running rife.

Those of us who want to do something about this weight gain try to do so by counting calories or cutting fat. Now we're getting even less sustenance from our food while still feeling exhausted and burned out all the time.

Now we feel guilty whenever we eat. Now our relationship with our food is even worse.

Scientists were very surprised when they looked at data from around the world and found that people who ate a Mediterranean Diet lived longer, were less likely to get heart disease and were thinner.

But when you think about it, it's obvious! These are people who spend actual time cooking fresh, healthy meals.

Many of those meals are PACKED with fruits, with vegetables, with salad and with fish. These are all foods that are stuffed with nutrients.

Nutrients that the body uses to build muscle, to regulate hormones, to provide energy and to improve our mood.

As soon as you start eating food that you enjoy – as soon as you slow down to smell the delicious garlic coming from your bolognaise – you begin eating well again and your body thanks you for it. Those living in the Mediterranean area have eaten this way for years and enjoy better health and more longevity than most in other areas ... there must be something to this way of living.

About the Author

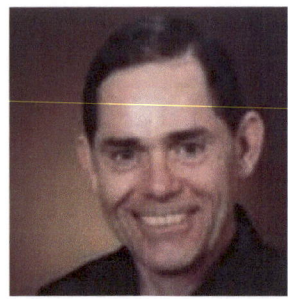

I have published over 125 books on Amazon for Kindle, CreateSpace and other publishing platforms.

While most of my books are on health and fitness in general, as I age (now 65) at the time of this writing) my topics of interest are geared toward aging baby boomers and older.

Besides my own writing, I also ghostwrite ebooks, books, reports, articles, blogs and do Kindle conversions for clients on a variety of topics.

Today my wife and I are retired from our careers and live in Gold Canyon, AZ. I now write as a retirement business where you'll find me happily sitting in my office typing away on my laptop as I work on my next book or ghostwriting project . . . that is if we are not traveling on a cruise ship - our new-found mode of travel.